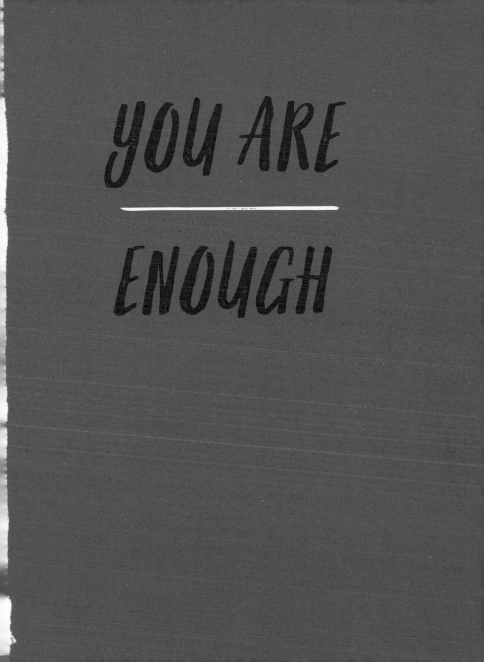

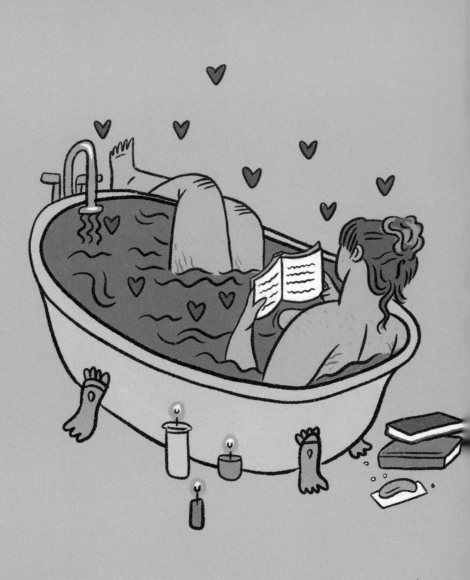

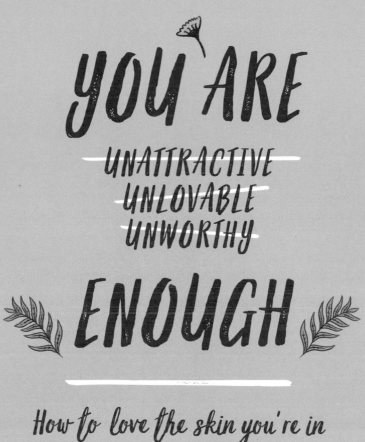

YOU ARE

~~UNATTRACTIVE~~

~~UNLOVABLE~~

~~UNWORTHY~~

ENOUGH

How to love the skin you're in
& embrace your awesomeness

Harri Rose

Illustrations by Ashley Lukashevsky

aster

An Hachette UK Company
www.hachette.co.uk

First published in Great Britain in 2019 by
Aster, an imprint of
Octopus Publishing Group Ltd
Carmelite House
50 Victoria Embankment
London EC4Y 0DZ
www.octopusbooks.co.uk
www.octopusbooksusa.com

Distributed in the US by
Hachette Book Group
1290 Avenue of the Americas
4th and 5th Floors
New York, NY 10104

Distributed in Canada by
Canadian Manda Group
664 Annette St.
Toronto, Ontario M6S 2C8

ISBN 978 1 78325 320 3

A CIP catalogue record for this book is
available from the British Library.

Printed and bound in China

10 9 8 7 6 5 4 3 2 1

Commissioned by: Emily Brickell
Art Director: Yasia Williams
Illustrator: Ashley Lukashevsky
Production Controller: Emily Noto
Photograph on page 112: Joe Lindsay

CONTENTS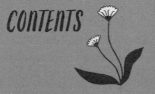

WHAT IS BODY ACCEPTANCE?

When it comes to how you feel about your body, I would put money on the claim that if I offered you a magic wand and said you could change it somehow, you'd jump at the chance. I say this because more than half the population is on some sort of "diet" at any one time, trying to shrink, buff, tone, lift and wish our bodies into a different shape.

It feels like every day there's a new quick fix to solve our body woes. It all sounds a bit like this out there:

+   ARE WE MEANT TO BE EATING FAT NOW?

+   CARBS ARE EVIL, YES?

+   DO CALORIES COUNT ANY MORE?

+   FRUIT IS FULL OF SUGAR, RIGHT?

+   WE'RE NOT MEANT TO EAT AT ALL FOR TWO DAYS A WEEK?!

+   THIS TEA IS GOING TO MAKE ME SKINNY! (DON'T TOUCH THAT TEA.)

+   PROTEIN, PROTEIN, PROTEIN?!

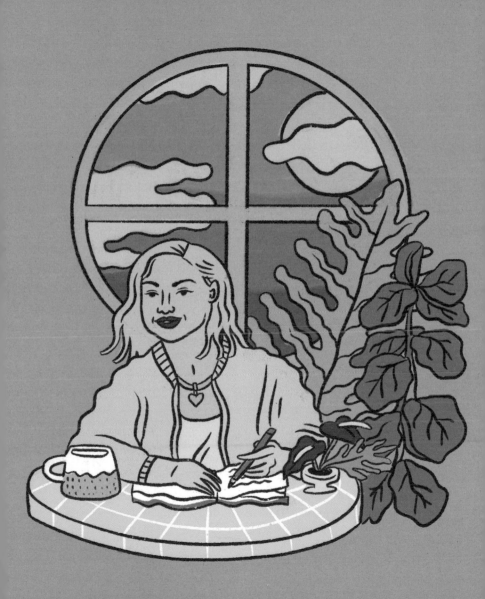

It's no wonder we've got no confidence around food and lost trust in our bodies to tell us how to feel good. Trust me, I used to be a walking dieting encyclopedia. Name a diet and I've tried it. I was obsessed with changing my body and spent years looking for "the one" (a diet to solve all my perceived problems, not a love match).

BUT HOLD TIGHT. THIS IS NOT A DIET BOOK. HELL NO! QUITE THE OPPOSITE.

What if this never-ending pursuit to change your body was a huge scam? What if I told you that within the pages of this book were ideas and exercises that could open your eyes to never wanting to change your body again? Hear me out.

I'm going to show you how it's possible to gain more freedom to enjoy your life than you can imagine right now.

How would I know? Because I coach people in unapologetic body acceptance. (Why unapologetic? Because for way too long we've been apologizing for our bodies! But don't worry, we'll get to that later.)

I've seen the changes that happen when people come off diets and find happiness within themselves. They go on to fill their lives with other things infinitely more interesting than plain grilled chicken and broccoli (hey, I'm not knocking it, I'm just saying no one asked for it as their last meal on earth).

This book, unlike many others, doesn't promise to make you thin. But it does hold the potential to make you happier in your body (which is good, because that magic wand I mentioned, it's pretty hard to come by).

I'll show you where to find the first steps on your own Yellow Brick Road out of negative body image and give you the tools (your own ruby slippers, if you will) that will not only help you start being kinder to yourself, but will also help you build healthy thoughts and habits that last. Things like: forget the gym if it feels like torture, but what about roller skating, wild swimming or sword fighting? *Newsflash* they're all good for your body.

KNOWING YOU ARE ENOUGH ISN'T ABOUT WHAT YOU LOOK LIKE, IT'S A MINDSET.

You don't have to wake up and love every inch of yourself every single day, every single minute. (I'm not building an army of narcissists here, nope.)

It means switching the focus from how you measure up on the outside to how you feel on the inside. And if you notice a negative thought about your body you're able to catch it, neutralize it and believe that you are more than worthy (which is kinda an ick word but it's useful because you are worthy) of living your best life, whatever this looks like for you (not just what Instagram says).

I want you to discover your own blend of what wellness looks like. That might be 6am yoga and green smoothies, but it very much might not be. It's about sometimes salads, sometimes mashed potato. You will not eat forever, I swear it, and I'll show you some practical tools to help you take back your power around food.

WHAT MAKES YOU FEEL GOOD WILL LOOK DIFFERENT FOR EVERYONE BECAUSE EVERY BODY IS DIFFERENT.

(Sorry, got a bit cheesy there, but true words.)

This journey isn't about thinking you're the most beautiful person on the planet, but rather believing that you deserve to live your best life *regardless* of what you look like. Just imagine how much freedom you're going to have when you're not spending every day fixated on food and wishing you looked different.

Imagine more adventures, more smiles, more struts down the beach, more laughter, more moments captured, more licks of the spoon, more colour, more sunshine on skin, more why nots, more shimmies on the dance floor thinking "I don't care how I look!" (and loving it) and more feeling like you're home (finally).

ARE YOU IN?...

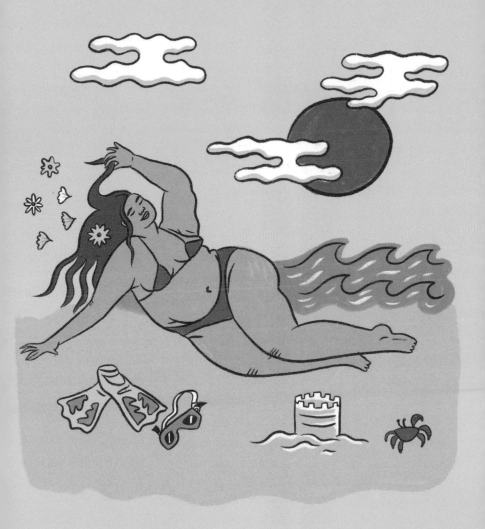

BREAKING FREE

In order to begin to fully own the awesomeness that is you, we have to begin with some understanding as to why so many of us are walking about doubting ourselves, hating our own reflections, comparing ourselves to strangers on the internet and wishing we looked entirely different. This chapter is about the world that we live in and why wanting to change the way we look is so tempting. It's also going to bust open all of those ideas, so hold onto your hats and keep an open mind, ok?

Here's a first activity to start seeing where you're at on the scale of liking yourself.

Grab a pen and a notebook, treat yourself to a new one if you like (mmm, new stationery – anyone else?) but don't let that stop you from just cracking on. Any bit of paper will do.

Ok, rate these statements from 1–10 (1 = hell no, big dislike; 5 = meh; 10 = all the yes, big like). Take a moment to ask yourself how you honestly feel about each of them, but don't overthink it. We'll come back to this at the end of the book.

+ **I CAN LOOK AT MYSELF NAKED IN THE MIRROR**

+ **I CAN LISTEN TO MY BODY TO TELL ME WHAT I NEED**

+ **I NEVER FEEL GUILTY ABOUT FOOD**

+ **I FEEL BODY CONFIDENT AROUND OTHERS**

+ **I FEEL COMFORTABLE IN MY OWN SKIN**

+ **I HAVE AN UNDERSTANDING OF WHAT DIET CULTURE MEANS AND THE IMPACT IT CAN HAVE**

+ **I CAN CATCH NEGATIVE THOUGHTS ABOUT MY BODY**

+ **I KNOW HOW TO BE KIND TO MYSELF**

Once you're done, take a minute to absorb the numbers, but don't despair if they're low. That's why you're here, right? Stay non-judgemental. This is super important. At this point, it's good to have a benchmark – by the time we're done, I'm confident you'll put all those numbers higher and be able to celebrate the mini-wins. **It's allllll about celebrating the mini-wins.**

WELCOME TO DIET CULTURE

This is a dystopian world where we must all strive to be thin in order to be happy... for our whole lives (no respite, Grandma). Where our other amazing skills, attributes and downright hilarious party tricks count far less than killer abs and a thigh gap (or, to be fair, simply whatever body type is *en vogue*).

Thin is the simple measure of beauty and success. We revere those people who magically "forget to eat", who still go to the gym even when they're really tired and who are able to say "no" to dessert every time.

> DIET CULTURE IS IN EVERY ADVERT, HOLLYWOOD MOVIE AND SNAPCHAT FILTER. BUT IT'S ALSO IN OUR SCHOOLS, WORKPLACES AND RELATIONSHIPS. IT SEEPS INTO THE CRACKS IN EVERY AREA OF OUR LIVES. IT'S EVERYWHERE AND IT'S INSIDIOUS.

If you're thin, diet culture says you've won at life. Ok, there's more to it than that, but currently society is engineered to cheer on those who fit this "thin ideal" (we'll talk more about the ridiculous one standard of beauty later) and berate those who don't measure up.

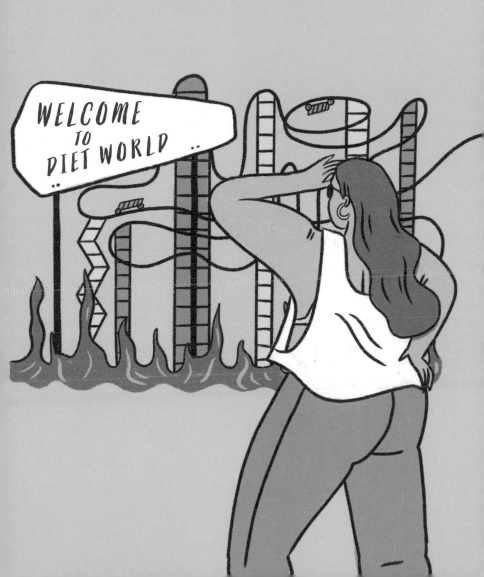

If you're fat, you must be lazy and eat too much, and therefore must go on a diet (pick any one) to become thin and worthy. This simple black-and-white thinking (based on the lies I'll chat about shortly) is diet culture.

IF THERE ARE RULES TO FOLLOW, IT'S A DIET, HONEY

For ease, let's put every self-esteem-bashing, body-image-crushing message we see under one umbrella term. Let's call it the diet industry because the end goal is always to change the way you look. If there are rules that dictate what you should be eating, then let's just call a spade a... diet.

The diet industry relies on – and makes some serious cha-cha-ching! from – us feeling bad about ourselves. The global diet industry is predicted to be worth more than $270 billion by 2023. That is one hellava lot of pounds being lost and found.

It preys upon our deepest insecurities and sells us future happiness. When one thing doesn't work, we blame ourselves, then move on to the next one, hoping this time, things will be different. And so the cycle continues.

DIET CULTURE IS SUPER SNEAKY

Diet culture is super sneaky, it gets into even the best of things. Even body positivity has gone from a small hashtag used to create a safe space on Instagram for people of colour and those in marginalized bodies to a huge movement. And have you searched that hashtag recently?

It's getting harder and harder to see the amazing people doing great things for marginalized bodies because it's now overrun with diet culture and people cashing in on its popularity, without a word to its origins.

Clothing companies are nodding to the rise of plus-size beauties without actually making their ranges inclusive. And you'll find all sorts of weight-loss BS like diet products, fitness programmes, waist trainers, booty lifters... you name it and I'll bet it's jumped on the body positivity bandwagon.

MYTHICAL PROBLEMS AND THE THINGS THAT FIX THEM

Here's a personal story about diet industry quackery that I'm sure is not uncommon. I once paid £100 ($125) for a woman to "infrared" my upper arms. I was promised that the red light would "blast my fat cells". I'm almost embarrassed to tell this story because it sounds so ludicrous, but that's how much I wanted to blast my bingos.

I may as well have burned my money (shocking, I know). When nothing had changed on the tape measure, the beauty therapist told me that I must not have changed my eating enough (erm, what was the light for then, love?!) and I left feeling ashamed and a failure. In reality, she pretty much stole my money and shamed me in the process.

> HOW MANY CRAZY THINGS HAVE YOU TRIED, OR PEOPLE IN YOUR LIFE TRIED IN THE PURSUIT OF THINNESS?

It's important to realize that any changes that happen to your body because of dieting won't automatically make you happy. This is because diets don't change your thoughts. I know because at my thinnest and fittest I was also the most messed up in the head. I never once really saw what I actually looked like.

Looking back, only in order to look forward

one
Make a list of all the things you've started or ways you've tried to change your body. Looking back can be painful, I feel you babe, just let whatever comes up pass through. We're only settling here for a moment so we can firm up our resolve for the future.

two
Think about how you felt or how old you were when you tried your first diet. Send some love to that version of yourself.

three
Know that you're doing your best, and always have been, and stay open to healing the relationship with your body. Because really, what is the likelihood that diet number 68 is "the one"?

four
Write a promise to yourself. "I, [your name], promise to stay open to the idea that I might not need to change my body to be happy. I promise to stay open to finding a new relationship with myself."

important side note
Look after yourself. Please don't look back if you know this is going to unearth some stuff you'd rather not look at. If this is the case, speak to a medical professional or see Resources on page 111.

WHY LOVE ISLAND ISN'T AS INNOCENT AS IT LOOKS

Let's take a moment to look at where beauty standards (the made-up rules telling us what is seen to be most attractive right now) show up A LOT.

I'm talking about reality television shows.

It doesn't matter which show you pick, the norm dictates that the cast be made up of under 25-year-old models and personal trainers, chosen specifically on their looks.

THE WORST THING ABOUT BEAUTY STANDARDS IS THAT THEY'RE ALWAYS CHANGING.

Currently, the beauty standard for a woman is to be thin and lightly toned with a big bum (#strongisthenewskinny) and for a man, the standard is to be lean with "abs for days". Yet, look back to the '90s and it was all bulky male muscles and female "heroine chic". The goal posts are *always* moving.

The problem – there are many problems, but one of the main ones is that the majority of the population will NEVER look like this. Thanks to genetics and a general lack of time and cash, the majority of us will be unable to craft ourselves into sculpted "sex symbols".

While these reality show cast members show off their bodies and their lifestyles, there are millions of people comparing their own bodies and feeling like they're coming up short.

Companies know this.

In the UK, one of the most popular shows of recent years is Love Island, with more than 4 million people regularly tuning in to watch a house full of singletons looking for love in the sunshine. In 2018, viewers who were streaming the show online (who are likely to be some of the youngest) were served up adverts for breast enlargements and diet pills. Seriously, WTAF.

So shocking were the adverts that it attracted criticism from the National Health Service and feminist groups, and thankfully the channel has agreed to review its advertising going forward.

But those companies chose to pay vast amounts of money for those slots, when viewers were likely to be comparing themselves to the contestants. And when we see a problem, they want to sell us a solution.

BEAUTY, FILLERS & FILTERS

Now, I luuuuurve a good lipstick. In my opinion, red lipstick is the warpaint that can make you feel 10-foot tall and able to take on any old ex you bump into at the bar. And what person would be against a great concealer that hides the fact you've only had two hours' sleep before rushing to get into the office? Nuh uh! Bring it on.

But we are contouring, shading and highlighting the f*** out of our faces like never before. And while there's nothing wrong with using makeup to make you feel good, there's a blurry line happening between beauty and the cosmetics industry.

And the power of celebrity to make us change our bodies and faces is **real**.

In 2015, Kylie Jenner confessed to having had lip fillers and it was reported that some clinics had a 70 per cent rise in enquiries. Since that initial announcement, Kylie has cashed in on lips. She created a multimillion-dollar company selling Kylie Lip Kits before expanding into Kylie Cosmetics. At the age of 21, Kylie became the world's youngest-ever billionaire.

While Botox and fillers used to be the hush-hush secret of women in their forties, more and more people in their twenties are seeking them out. There are even reports of Snapchat facial dysmorphia, where we lose perspective of what a normal face should look like.

> THE REASON FOR THIS RISE IN COSMETIC PROCEDURES IS THIS SINGLE STANDARD OF BEAUTY. WE ARE TOLD THERE'S ONLY ONE WAY TO BE BEAUTIFUL.

Yet, have you ever met a person who didn't have nice eyes? No! Faces are amazing! They don't need changing.

One of the most beautiful things about human beings is the diversity of our faces – noses, lips, eyes, ears – all different shapes and sizes. Wouldn't it be so boring if we all suddenly had to look the same?

In 2018, Kylie Jenner reportedly removed all of her fillers – just think about that before you book a procedure. Fashion changes. But your face is yours forever.

YOU AREN'T FAILING DIETS, DIETS ARE FAILING YOU

Ok, let's get out of diet world for a moment, which by now I hope you'll see is an absolute house of horrors for our body image. Time to look at the reasons why diets are so tempting and what they actually do to your body.

Here's the truth: diets do not work in the long term. There is a heap of research to back this up.

Fact: 95–98 per cent of diets fail, with two-thirds of people putting the weight back on and sometimes more, within three years (see Michael Hobbes's HuffPost article, "Everything You Know About Obesity Is Wrong").

Millions of pounds are being pumped into research about why the world is getting bigger. And while there's talk around lifestyle factors, increased chemicals and even the bacteria in our guts, there's still no magic pill (or shake, tea or meal) that's going to make us thin (regardless of which shiny celebrity might be fronting it). If there was, we'd probably all be taking it, because we all know the world is a much easier place for those who don't worry about their weight.

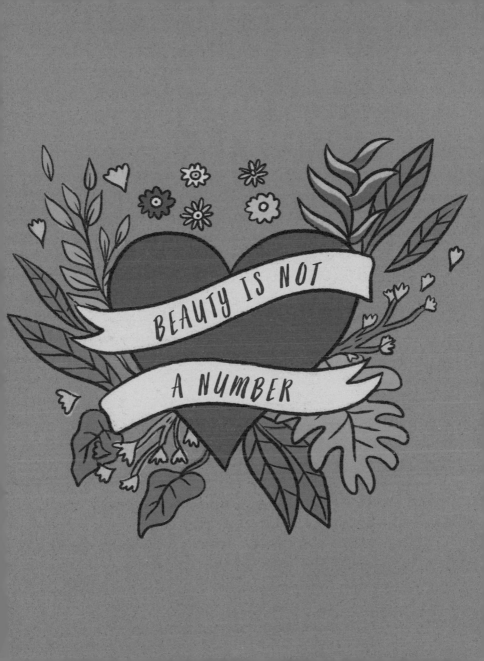

Here are a few things we know about how the human body reacts to diets:

+ **EVOLUTION IS SMART**
  We have a genetic weight set point that's really difficult to move away from. The body wants to keep weight on as a survival mechanism, so there's a lot of resistance when we try to change it. We're usually able to move 10–20lbs either side but each body knows what size it wants to be and will fight to get it back. (*Newsflash* it might not be a size 6.)

+ **METABOLISM IS A BITCH**
  The more we diet, the more we mess up our internal regulation system. Restrictive diets actually slow down your metabolism (yes really!) and it never recovers, even when you start eating more food again. That means you're more likely to have put *on* weight since starting dieting. (WTAF, right? I told you diets were evil.)

+ **WILLPOWER IS LIMITED**
  Diets rely on willpower and this, by its very nature, is limited. Therefore, diets are almost impossible to maintain long term. Not only that, what happens when we tell ourselves we can't have something? We want it MORE. The body is clever: when you're restricting, your body is sending you hunger hormones so you feel the need to eat more.

+ **IT'S A SLIPPERY SLOPE**
  Diets are heavily linked to disordered eating as this struggle between physical needs versus mental willpower can lead to binge eating behaviours and sometimes eating disorders. If you've ever gone from having an extra nibble

to full-blown, out-of-control flood of eating whatever food you can get your hands on, then you've potentially fallen into a "f*** it window". This is where you feel you've blown your diet so you may as well eat EVERYTHING before you start again, usually on Monday. This triggers even more feelings of shame and failure. But it's not your fault! Diets send us all round the bend because they mess with us mentally as well as physically.

There's even evidence that "yo-yo dieting" can lead to pretty scary health issues, such as increased risk of diabetes, high blood pressure, hypertension, stroke and coronary heart disease.

YET SOCIETY SAYS THAT IT'S OUR FAULT WE CAN'T CHANGE OUR BODIES (GOOD ONE SOCIETY *EYE ROLL*) AND BECAUSE OUR SOCIAL MEDIA FEED IS FULL OF SUCCESSFUL-LOOKING "BEFORE-AND-AFTER" PHOTOS WE THINK THERE MUST BE SOMETHING WRONG WITH US

Quite frankly, this is complete BS. You're fighting biology.

At the very least, dieting is a waste of time and energy. At its worst it can ruin lives through eating disorders. I wish I had always known what I do now, because it would have saved me a ton of tears and years of my own disordered relationship with food and my body. But do not despair. **I'm going to show you a different path to loving yourself, I promise.**

BUT WHAT ABOUT WELLNESS?

Ah yes, wellness. Ok, there is absolutely nothing wrong with wanting to look after your health. Showing an interest in what's on your plate is deffo a good thing. It's obviously s*** tons (technical measure) better to eat a diet rich in quinoa than the 1990s crash diets of grapefruit and black coffee.

Let's get real here. "Wellness" is often diet culture dressed in fancy Lycra. It lures you with expensive, exotic-sounding ingredients like moringa and baobab. Have you met anyone who actually enjoys the taste of spirulina or wheatgrass?

IF THERE'S SOMEONE TELLING YOU HOW BEST TO EAT FOR YOUR BODY, IT'S A DIET. PLAIN AND SIMPLE.

These days, wellness is just health with a price tag. As Ruby Tandoh says in her book *Eat Up*, "The way to upper-middle-class white girl heaven? You gotta get there through chia seeds, suppressing all your natural urges, and yoga."

"Wellness warriors" (often thin, white, privileged women) sell us aspirational living. The more we control our bodies and the more expensive the gym membership, the more successful we are seen to be.

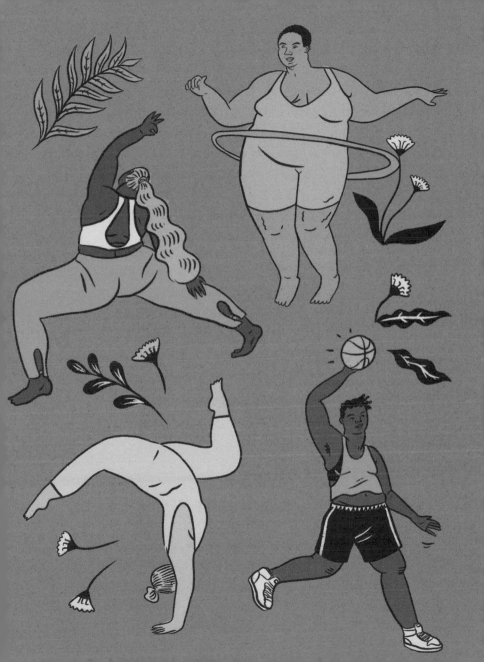

As millennials have less money than previous generations, "health" is the new social capital. Being thin (or toned, ripped, built or whatever gym body you're going for) has become more than just body shape. It has become a status symbol. Being able to buy organic vegetables, expensive supplements and a personal trainer now gets the same nod of approval as buying a big house used to, and arguably those without are seen to be less worthy. This is BS.

Let's break it down. Not everyone will learn to do a handstand or make a smoothie bowl. Not everyone can afford to exercise anywhere apart from the local park or in their home. Not everyone can buy their shopping at Waitrose. But you know what? Tinned tomatoes were once on the vine too.

What happened to throwing on an old T-shirt you don't mind getting gross and sweaty in for exercise? Now it's like you can't possibly enter a gym unless you're rocking a full outfit that you'd also be able to wear to brunch. It's ridic.

True wellbeing isn't about how little cellulite you have or if you can make a cauliflower into a "pizza". There are no prizes for how expensive your leggings are and no wonder ingredient that will stop us all from dying. Sorry to be blunt, but it's true.

Beware the people with shiny hair telling you to seek expensive ingredients to "be well". And run in the opposite direction of anyone giving it large about detox: they are talking nonsense. Your body does a damn fine job of detoxing via your inbuilt detox pixies (cheers liver and kidneys, you rock).

MEASURING YOUR WORTH BY THE WRONG SCALE

Incredible people like you are wasting their whole lives not embracing how f*ing magical they are, right now.**

Your body, with its 37 trillion cells (!), is doing its darndest to keep you alive throughout your lifetime. (Yeah John Mayer, "Your Body is a Wonderland" is not just your slightly creepy song, but biological FACT). You are so much more than a number, you are made of stardust don't you know?

By living by the scales (or Fitbit or macros, whatever gadget is God right now), you are shrinking your worth and happiness into a digit. Unless you have a medical reason for checking the micro-biology of your being, I propose another path. (Like, *how do you actually feel in your body?* But we'll get on to that.)

Let's take a moment. Picture your best friend right now.

Put them at the front of your mind, let all the memories of the best times you've had together flash past. Think about their smile, their laugh, their funny expressions and all of the reasons that you love them. (Now send them a message to tell them you love them, just because it's a nice thing to do and we don't do it enough. Then come back to the book.)

So, how does that relate to the work we're doing here? Well, in that daydream, did you at any point think, "Oh man, I love how dedicated to the gym Suzie is" or, "I really dig the sculpted shape of Nadya's calves" or, "I cannot get over how awesomely Jemima can follow food rules"?

I doubt it.

No. You remembered that time they goofed about so much you almost wet yourself. Or when they stood up for you, or perhaps the times they've held back your hair (true love, right there) or simply held your hand as you cried.

> YOU DON'T LOVE PEOPLE FOR THE SHELLS THEY RESIDE IN. YOU LOVE THEM FOR THE QUALITIES THEY POSSESS. THE CHARACTERISTICS THEY ADMIRE AND THEIR DOGGED DETERMINATION TO SEE THE BEST IN YOU, JUST AS YOU DO IN THEM BECAUSE: THAT IS LOVE.

So what the hell do you do in this zombie apocalypse wasteland for body confidence? **You have to be a rebel and learn to embrace the skin you're in.** And let's get one thing straight – this does not mean giving up. (Louder for those at the back: IT IS NOT GIVING UP.)

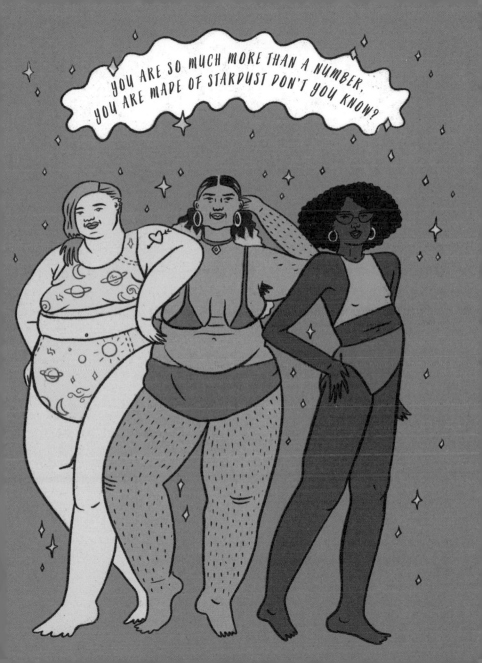

99 problems, but your body ain't 1

Because you may have ninety-nine problems but you're about to learn that you and your body ain't one of them. This activity isn't meant to be easy, but you can do it.

one

Remember that little daydream we had about our best friend?

two

Write down all the tiny things that your best friend might say about you.

Find a piece of paper and go!

three

Running out of things? Think about all the amazing ways that your body keeps you alive, e.g. your heart is beating, your lungs are breathing...

four

Send some gratitude (say thank you) to all of your amazing characteristics and incredible things about your body (that don't rely on you looking a certain way).

Research shows that when we spend time feeling grateful, it improves our mental health and our self-esteem.

WHY BODY ACCEPTANCE ISN'T GIVING UP

When I tell people what I do for a living they automatically assume that by learning to be kind to yourself and listening to your body, you'll stop wanting to eat healthy food, stop exercising and never leave your sofa. *face-palm* This could not be further from the truth.

I want you to be one of the people who loves their body regardless of how much, or not at all, it changes. I want you to see that you are lovable at every stage of your existence because you are way more than your body.

> SAYING "I THINK I'M PRETTY DAMN FINE!" AND
> LIKING IT, WOW, THAT'S HUGE.

Just imagine how much more time and brain space you'll have when you're not worrying so much about what you look like. Body acceptance isn't giving up, it's freedom. When you can begin to feed your body kindness, it's amazing what you'll discover. And new is good because old wasn't working.

★ SUMMARY ★

+ WE LIVE IN A SOCIETY THAT SAYS BEING THIN IS THE MOST IMPORTANT THING YOU CAN BE. THIS IS CALLED DIET CULTURE AND WE NEED TO REBEL AGAINST THIS.

+ THE DIET INDUSTRY (WHICH IS IN EVERYTHING) IS PROFITING FROM YOUR INSECURITIES.

+ DIETS DO NOT WORK. FACT. THEY MESS UP YOUR BODY AND YOUR MIND.

+ YOU ARE WAY MORE THAN YOUR BODY. TIME TO STOP MEASURING YOUR WORTH BY A NUMBER ON A SCALE.

+ LEARNING TO ACCEPT YOUR BODY IS FREEDOM TO HAVE AND DO MORE THAN YOU CAN IMAGINE. IT IS NOT GIVING UP.

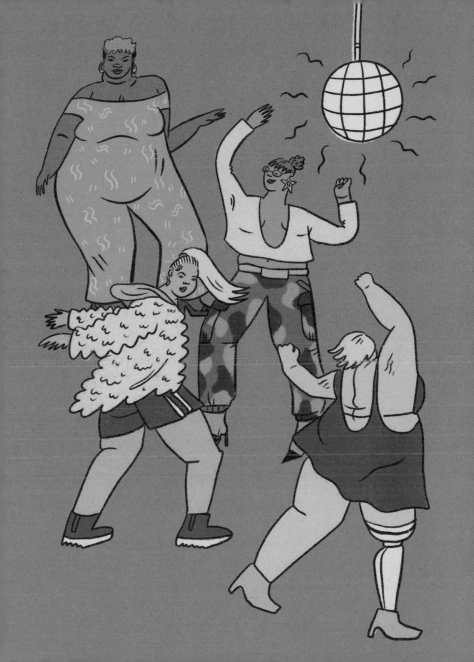

LEARNING TO MAKE PEACE WITH FOOD & YOUR BODY

By now you're probably thinking "hold on a minute, is this one of those self-love books?" Well, you got me: this is a path to loving yourself. But before you throw down these pages and walk away, I'm not about to leap into lists about baths bombs, candles and how you just need to mouth "I love you" in the mirror.

For loads of people, the idea of "loving themselves" is a super cheesy concept (honestly, I get it). And it can feel like such a long way from where you're at, that it's easy to dismiss it as "fine for them but not for me".

YET IT'S VERY DIFFICULT TO HATE YOURSELF INTO SELF-LOVE (WHICH IS ESSENTIALLY WHAT DIETS SUGGEST YOU CAN DO).

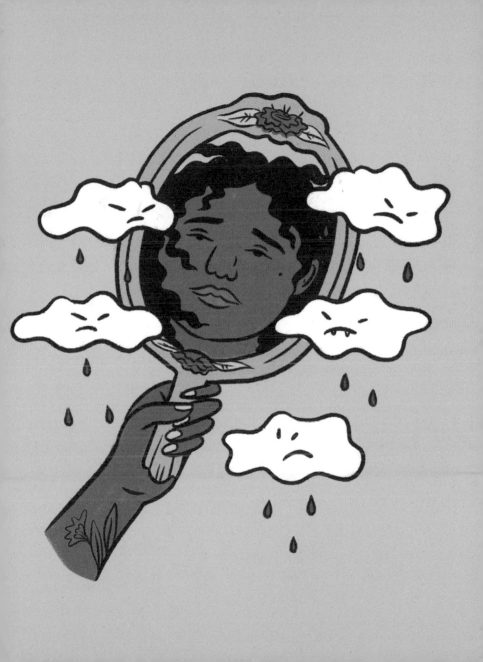

YOUR BODY HEARS EVERYTHING YOUR BRAIN TELLS IT

When I first heard this expression, it hit me pretty hard. Too often we cut ourselves off at the neck – we don't mind our faces, but wish we could have a full-body switch-up.

But when we're saying, "I hate my chin", "I hate my legs", "I hate my back" – we don't realize that we're throwing stones at ourselves. We *are* the school bully.

> I DIDN'T WANT TO BE AT WAR WITH MYSELF,
> BUT I'D BEEN SO ON AUTOPILOT THAT I HADN'T
> REALIZED THAT MY INNER WORLD WAS AS BRUTAL
> AS THE OUTER ONE.

The most crushing thing is, your body has been taking it all this time. Not holding judgment, not wishing your brain into oblivion (which, quite frankly, it would be entitled to do). Nope. Your body has been silently, patiently waiting for you to stop the insults, the verbal punches and the tantrums – and come home. But we'll get to that.

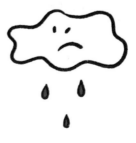

BODY NEUTRALITY WAVING THE WHITE FLAG

A concept that's super useful if you and your body have been sworn nemeses since totes forever is "body neutrality".

This is the space in which you can wave a white flag and draw up a peace treaty between you and your body. It's a time for reconnecting while still giving yourself permission to feel *all the feels*. And it's where you and your body can sit across the table from each other, suss each other out and shake hands.

It's a really important phase and one that can be neglected in the world of "Instagrammable" and "Pinterestable" "self-love" (that's a hellava lot of inverted commas).

Importantly, there will be some people who feel getting to a neutral place is a perfectly respectable end goal. If you're one of those, then no shame here. Meet yourself where you are and know that baby steps are totally cool in this work.

WHERE TO BEGIN...

Try the Shining a Light on the Slime activity (see pages 42–45) to hear how critical the voice you've been using against yourself is. From here you'll start creating a kinder, more neutral stance. Neutral thoughts are pretty magical because they can see both the negative and positive but not take a side. They stay impartial and non-judgemental. The Switzerland of thoughts, if you will.

Shining a light on the slime

This activity is like shining a light into the dark,
dank cave bits of our brain. This is where the thoughts
we never share with anyone else live and where our
inner bitch lurves to stockpile her ammo.

What we're doing here is starting to become an observer
(a nice one, not a creepy one) of the things we're telling
ourselves and look at them in a non-judgemental way.

Sometimes, with our thoughts, we internalize
the nasty things someone says to us and use them
against ourselves (we all do this, don't worry). For
example, if someone made a body comment about
your legs at the age of 16, you might still use that
comment against yourself at the age of 26. Not only
do these thoughts hold us back they also keep
a divide (or a war) between us and our bodies.

And by keeping these thoughts in our heads, and
not telling anyone about them, they can grow in power
and leave us feeling "icky" (another technical term)
and embarrassed. This feeling can be called shame -
and it lurves secrecy. (For more on this check out
Brené Brown's amazing work, it's game changing).

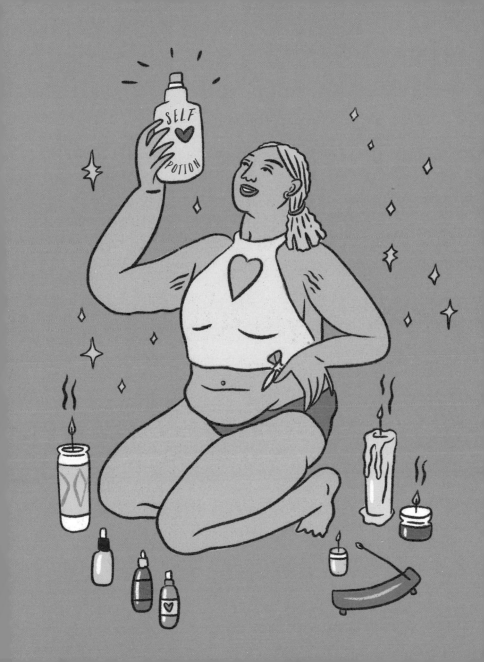

Time to stop shaming ourselves with these stories.

By creating space between ourselves and these slimy thoughts, we're able to begin to take away their sting - and eventually let them go.

Please note that if at any time you want to stop that's totally OK. This stuff is deeeeeep. Self-care is key.

one
Write down the list of means thoughts you say to yourself. Try and stay non-judgemental. Just observe the thoughts as if you're listening to the radio. Be curious. Label it for what it is - simply a thought.

two
Read back and reflect. Read the sentences back but replace any "you are" sentences with "I am" and change any "your" to "my". So for example, "You are fat and lazy" becomes "I am fat and lazy". Take a moment to realize these are words you probably wouldn't use against your worst enemy and it's time to stop using them against yourself.

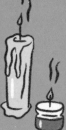

three

Neutral reframe. Noticing our thoughts and labelling
them is a great first step to healing. For some extra oomph!
try writing a neutral statement for each negative thing
you wrote above. This is an opportunity to reframe from how
your body looks to what it can do and how it can make you
feel. e.g. "my stomach helps me digest food" or "my boobs are
a natural part of my body" or "my legs help me feel strong"

four

Practice, practice, practice. It's ok if this is hard -
reprogramming the way we've been talking to ourselves
for years can take a long time.

important side notes

Remember, it's not about how well your body functions.
For those with disability, chronic pain or disease, I know
this exercise is hard. Please know that your body's ability
to function doesn't increase or decrease your worth on this
planet. Your body will be doing the best that it can - just
saying that can be healing in creating a kinder inner dialogue.

Mindfulness is a great practical tool for learning how
to observe and be non-judgemental about your thoughts.
I highly recommend the Headspace App if you want an easy
way into learning more about this.

YOU ARE AS MUCH YOUR THIGHS AS YOUR EYES

In my work I've found that most people have no problem saying they like their eyes, but find it incredibly easy to pick apart other areas of their body. But hunny, it's all you! When you see that you are as much your thighs as your eyes, big shifts happen. This is the start of seeing yourself as the whole of your parts. Then the healing can really begin.

WTF IS INTUITIVE EATING & WHY YOU WON'T EAT FOREVER

"But what about food?" I hear you cry. If you're anything like my clients, you probably feel like you can't be trusted around food. You likely feel that if you let go of your rules, then you'll never stop eating. You might even think that there's something wrong with you because you're fixated on food and can't stop thinking about it. All. The. Time.

I promise you, this is not true.

When babies are born they have in-built wisdom that tells them when they need food and when they've had enough. They eat from a place of intuition. They don't think about it. You also popped out into the world with this power. You weren't born over-analysing the calorific content of milk, apple puree or [insert your favourite baby munch here].

The glorious news is, you can take this power back again! Yes, it involves being brave and trusting that you have the knowledge to eat in a way that makes you feel good. If it feels scary to think about letting go of the rule book, then know you're not alone. This can be a big step. But YOU CAN DO IT.

BUT WHAT IF IT'S NOT HEALTHY?

If you're forever "trying to be good", why are there times when "healthy food" never quite hits the spot? When I was trapped in dieting, there were times when all I wanted was a piece of toast, but I wasn't "allowed" bread so I'd eat something "good" like celery. When that didn't do it, I'd "allow myself" a diet crispbread or two (probably with cottage cheese – I used to buy family-size tubs of it). And so the munching would continue. Down the list of my allowed "healthy foods" I'd chomp, until I'd have eaten far more than if had I simply given myself permission to eat the toast in the first place.

WHAT ARE YOU HUNGRY FOR?

Many of us aren't eating from a place of nourishment. Nourishment, of course, is giving your body the right types of foods to function optimally (nutritionally living your best life). But in reality, food is much more than the sum of its parts.

Food is also about pleasure, comfort, community, a mix of grab-what's-available, plan something-for-hours and a lot in between – from impulse-buy samosas, 4pm squares of chocolate at your desk, last of the pay cheque/last of the fridge mash-ups, to break-up brownies, home-cooked dinners with the girls served with (large) glasses of white wine and a "ta da!", date-night pizza, family roasts and celebration feasts.

We eat for a multitude of reasons, hunger being one of them. It's incredibly normal to want to eat your heartbreak away or run your finger round an empty plate that once held something so delicious you're genuinely sad it's over.

DIETING RUINS FOOD MEMORIES

When you throw a diet mentality into the mix, your relationship with food experiences becomes conditional. A series of: Am I "allowed" this? How often can I show up for this? What will happen at the scales if I eat this?

Each food moment is balanced somewhere between "I shouldn't" and "f*** it". And is often followed by guilt, shame, restriction and potentially more "f*** its" if you feel you've blown it and will start again tomorrow (or Monday).

> DIET RULES MAKE FOOD A BATTLE. A SLOG. THEY TAKE AWAY THE PLEASURE AND DISCONNECT US FROM WHAT EATING FROM A PLACE OF TRUE NOURISHMENT REALLY FEELS LIKE. THIS IS WHY FOOD IS SO TRICKY AND WHY RE-LEARNING HOW TO EAT CAN BE SO HARD.

Eat when you're hungry and stop when you're full is never that easy if you've had a #itscomplicated relationship with eating. (On a serious note, if you've been diagnosed with an eating disorder in the past, then please reach out to a medical professional. See Resources on page 111 for more information.)

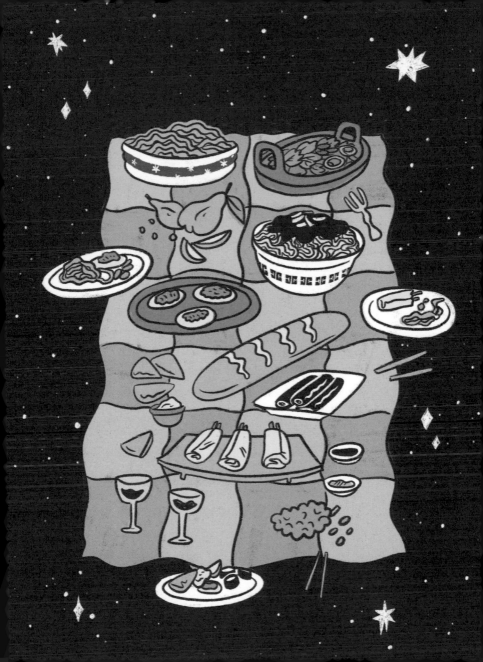

Here is a list of things that food doesn't need to be:

+ It doesn't need to be eaten in secret, in the dark or in the car - or when everyone else has gone to bed.

+ It doesn't need to be something that speaks to you from inside wrappers and boxes so loudly that you cannot have it in the house for fear of eating every morsel.

+ It doesn't have to be "being good" for five days and "naughty" for two in a weekly cycle of extremes.

+ It doesn't have to be grazing throughout the evenings not knowing how to stop.

+ It doesn't have to be wanting to order one thing but feeling peer-pressured to order something else "more healthy".

+ It doesn't have to be pride in saying "no" to it.

+ It doesn't have to be guilt at saying "yes".

+ It doesn't have to be shameful or something you can fail at.

+ It doesn't have to be difficult.

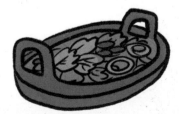

Here's how eating expert Ellyn Satter sums it up so concisely:

"Normal eating is going to the table hungry and eating until you are satisfied. It is being able to choose food you like and eat it and truly get enough of it - not just stop eating because you think you should. Normal eating is being able to give some thought to your food selection so you get nutritious food, but not being so wary and restrictive that you miss out on enjoyable food. Normal eating is giving yourself permission to eat sometimes because you are happy, sad or bored, or just because it feels good. Normal eating is mostly three meals a day, or four or five, or it can be choosing to munch along the way. It is leaving some cookies on the plate because you know you can have some again tomorrow, or it is eating more now because they taste so wonderful. Normal eating is overeating at times, feeling stuffed and uncomfortable. And it can be undereating at times and wishing you had more. Normal eating is trusting your body to make up for your mistakes in eating. Normal eating takes up some of your time and attention, but keeps its place as only one important area of your life. In short, normal eating is flexible. It varies in response to your hunger, your schedule, your proximity to food and your feelings."

Quote reproduced with permission from *Secrets of Feeding a Healthy Family: How to Eat, How to Raise Good Eaters, How to Cook* by Ellyn Satter

I believe that the key word in that paragraph is **"choose"**.

+ **WHEN YOU CHOOSE HOW TO EAT CONSCIOUSLY, IT PUTS YOU BACK IN CONTROL.**

+ **CHOOSING HELPS YOU DECIDE WHAT TO EAT AND HOW MUCH, IN ORDER TO FEEL SATISFIED.**

+ **CHOOSING STOPS BINGES AND INCREASES MINDFULNESS.**

+ **CHOOSING IS POWER.**

The problem is that we have a society that is set up to sell us food at every opportunity (notice just how much chocolate there is at every checkout these days), then slams us for eating it. (Big food companies + diet culture = evil genius.)

We think we're choosing when we go on a diet or put rules in place, but that's giving the power to external forces. We have to learn how to trust our bodies again. And we have to learn to work *with* our bodies rather than against them. We have to choose to get to know ourselves again.

You still have the natural dashboard of internal intelligence that you were born with. Sure, it might have been taking a battering (or a sledge hammering) while you've been restricting all these years. It'll probably need a bit of a tune-up. But it's there. **I told you, bodies are magic.**

THE MAGICAL TOOL OF INTUITIVE EATING

The original book, *Intuitive Eating* by Evelyn Tribole and Elyse Resch, goes much deeper into this topic than can be crammed between these short pages. But let's take a zip through some of the fundamentals so you can start to lay the foundations. (Remember that Yellow Brick Road to happiness I told you about? Well, this Is definitely one of the biggest steps on it.)

Step one on an intuitive eating journey is to reject diet mentality. Hopefully by now you'll have started to see diet culture as the BS that it is, so let's get into the practicalities of how to eat.

Learning how to eat again takes practice and a lot of attention. IT'S NOT EASY. Although we only have time to skip over these steps, please hear me, I know this isn't a walk in the park. You may well think, "Harri Rose this is boring and tedious and makes me feel like I'm an alien in my own body." But please stick with it. All the food moments I talked about earlier get a lot easier to navigate once you're back in tune with your body. Just. Keep. Going. You can do it.

SOME FOUNDATIONS TO GET YOU STARTED

+ **GET TO KNOW YOUR HUNGER**

+ **EAT WHAT YOU'RE HUNGRY FOR**

+ **STOP WHEN YOU'RE FULL**

+ **EAT FROM A PLACE OF JOY**

GET TO KNOW YOUR HUNGER

Get curious about where hunger sits in your body. Is it in your stomach? Is it under your rib cage? It is in your throat? It is noises or a feeling? Does your mood change? ("I'm so sorry for what I said when I was hangry." This is me.)

Not sure? Then wait. Eventually you'll get a picture – almost like a sliding scale of messages from your body. When exploring this, please don't allow yourself to get so hungry that you're shaking or numbed out.

There are now no rules except that when you're hungry you're allowed to eat. Simple. Regardless of the time of day or how much you've already eaten. Your body needs food. So eat.

EAT WHAT YOU'RE HUNGRY FOR

This is important, so please hear me when I say... YOU MUST EAT WHATEVER AND HOWEVER MUCH YOU WANT. Yep, if you fancy it, dig in – chocolate cake, pasta, pancakes, cheese on toast, cookies or mini quiche. Your job is to tune in and have a conversation with your belly. Your body knows best.

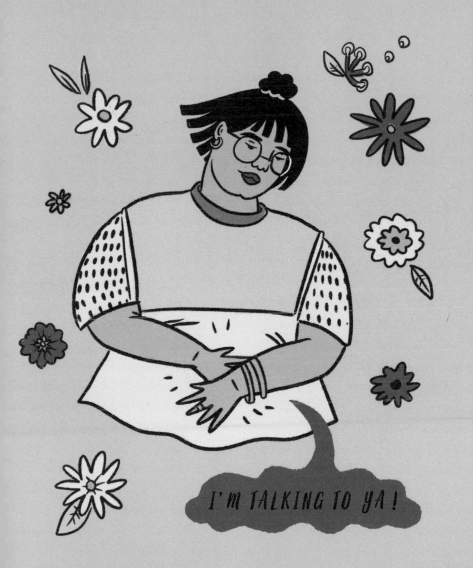

"Bad foods" are the ones we're never allowed to eat. We tell ourselves they're *extra* tempting and we cannot be controlled around them (like a wild woman, no crumb would be safe). But it's the restriction that triggers binges, not the food itself.

Eating what you want will be scary. Push through the fear and all the thoughts that shout that food rules are needed for you to be happy and healthy. After a while, you'll no longer feel the need to eat it. I promise you, no body wants to live on chocolate cookies forever.

Eventually your body will say "Please can I have a salad or a plate of broccoli?". Your body wants to be well and intuitively you'll discover that comes from eating a range of different foods. When you stop associating healthy foods with dieting, you'll discover what makes you feel most alive. You may even find you start craving spinach. For realz.

STOP WHEN YOU'RE FULL

Now you're eating from a place of no rules, you can tell your body that there'll always be enough. This means there's no need to overeat when food is around – and that makes stopping a whole lot easier.

We demonize fullness because diets celebrate hunger – but hear me hunny, fullness is your friend. Fullness is your body saying "Cheers love! I've had enough for now". It doesn't mean you've overeaten. It's a totally normal signal from your body. Eat slowly, keep checking in, noticing and, when you feel satisfied, practise stopping. It won't always be easy. Stay kind.

EATING FROM A PLACE OF JOY

When you choose foods that make you smile and make you feel happy, then you'll feel more satisfied.

You deserve to eat in a way that makes you feel good. You deserve to eat food that makes you say yum. This doesn't need to be a three-course dinner (hello, reality), but you deserve to eat without misery, fear, guilt, shame or secrecy.

There's nothing wrong with loving food. You don't need a *newsflash* to know that food is delicious. Only diet culture makes us think we're wrong for salivating and savouring and having full bellies. Eat food that brings you joy.

For a deep dive into intuitive eating, check out the original book by Evelyn Tribole and Elyse Resch, listed in Further Reading (see page 110).

SIDE NOTE: EMOTIONAL EATING IS NORMAL

Sometimes it's easier to eat our feelings because food is comfort. But it's important to spend some time working out why you want to eat if you aren't hungry. Are you tired, anxious, sad or frustrated? Can you call a friend, ask for help, go for a walk, even shout or have a cry instead? If there's no solution, see if you can sit with the feeling. Be kind to yourself. Your mental health is important and you deserve to be treated with kindness. Self-care isn't about bubble baths, it takes massive balls to ask for your needs to be met.

WHAT'S MINDFULNESS GOT TO DO WITH IT?

We eat with the telly on, phone in hand, chatting to others. We eat thinking about our work problems, family life and pretty much focus on everything else except what we're putting in our mouths. When we're distracted, we're eating on autopilot. We're not tasting, we're not savouring and we're not being present enough to listen to our bodies and ask ourselves "How does this food make me feel?".

Try the Mindful Eating activity (see pages 60–61) to learn what it means to eat mindfully. Although it's not realistic to think we all have hours in the day to switch everything off and focus directly on our plates, try to do this as often as you can. Could you set a target of one meal a day? The more mindful we can be, the more we can assess what foods make us feel most well.

YOU GET TO DECIDE HOW TO EAT

It's important you know that no one eats mindfully and intuitively all the time. The principles of intuitive eating are just tools so that YOU get to decide when and how to eat.

So you get to decide whether you want dessert on a date or whether or not to partake in Susan's birthday cake at work, or if you fancy porridge or leftover curry for breakfast.

You get to make the rules. And you get to decide when and what is right for your body.

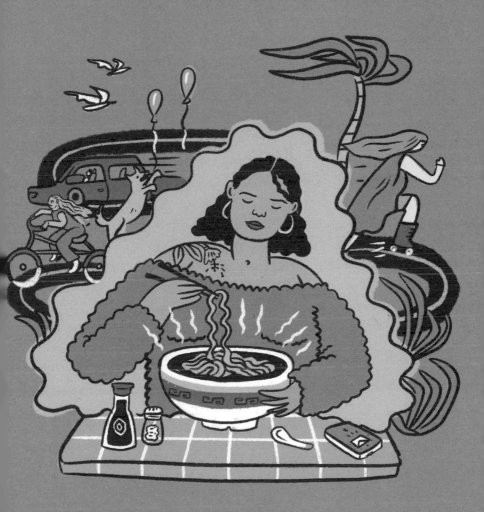

Mindful eating

Find a time when you can eat without distraction. The reason for this exercise is that the more we can be present when we eat, the more we can make choices that satisfy us. Not only that, but when we're able to tune in and listen to our bodies, the easier it gets to hear when we've had enough. It's pretty hard work at first but it gets easier, I promise.

one
Before this exercise, choose something you really fancy to eat. I've been recommended chocolate, raisins and olives as good options. My preference is chocolate (but then I love chocolate!). There are no rules, no good or bad. Just pick something you like.

two
Sit down. Put away your phone. Turn off the TV. Close that book. (We're getting present here.) Close your eyes for a few minutes and take a few breaths. Try to feel what it feels like to be in your body right now. Feel your lungs expanding, feel your belly rise and fall. Spend a few moments here.

three

When you are ready, look at your chosen item
with curiosity. What do you notice? How does it feel?
How does it smell? Is there a pattern to it?
Just notice.

four

Ok, so we're going to eat it now, but when you
put it in your mouth, don't swallow it instantly.
Allow it to just melt or dissolve. What's the texture like?
Is it hot, cold, spicy, soft, crunchy? Do you like the taste?
Reeeeeeally focus on the sensations.

five

When you're ready, swallow.
What did you learn? When we begin to listen it's amazing
what we start to discover. How does your mouth feel now?
How does your body feel? Could you be more present
for a whole meal? What would that look like? Begin to see
how much more you could get from your food experiences
by being more present and mindful.

LOSS OF THE DREAM

Such a huge part of body acceptance is grieving your "fantasy body". You know the one – the one you've had as a poster in your mind forevs. Your "dream body", which makes all your problems disappear!

I know how it feels to daydream over transformation photos, wishing (more than anything) to look like that.

Imagining a future when you'll be thin/toned/sculpted and be able to frolic naked, free from insecurity. Or buying clothes too small as "motivation" for your future body. Ugh. These things need to stop.

It's time to let it go. Letting go can be painful, full of despair and loss of hope. However, it's important to acknowledge this as part of the process.

TRUTHFULLY, THE BODY YOU HAVE NOW IS MORE THAN WORTHY OF LOVE, KINDNESS AND ACCEPTANCE.

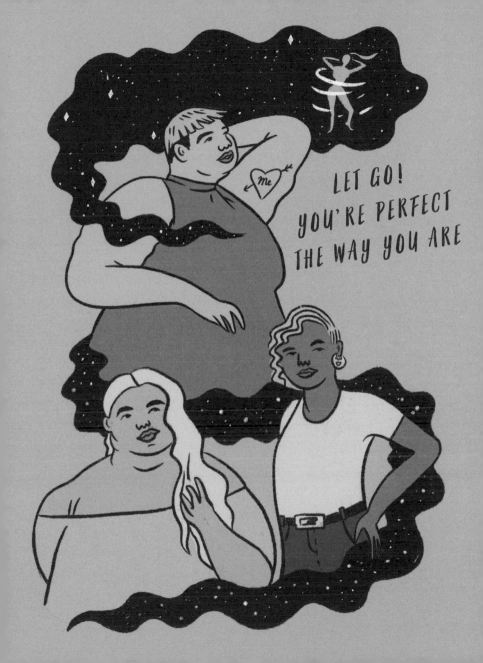

Remember that it's only diet culture that says we're all meant to look the same. It's only the media that shows us one body of "worth" on our screens, and the beauty industry that tells us there's only one way to be beautiful.

> THIS BODY IS THE ONLY ONE YOU'LL EVER HAVE.
> YOU MAY AS WELL LEARN TO BE FRIENDS WITH
> IT, RIGHT?!

Letting go of a future imagined body is hard. But please don't think this means you'll never change. It isn't the end of happiness. It's the start of freedom, remember? (Don't worry, we're going to get much more into this in the next chapter.)

When we let go of an idea that has been holding us back, we create space for a new reality to emerge.

This work isn't easy. And as I've said before, self-love in a hard world is courageous. You'll need to have a rebel heart, but I believe in you.

Visualizing the loss of the fantasy body

This exercise needs a pen, paper and some time when you can use your imagination. We're all busy, so carve out 15-30 mins and revisit the visualization as often as you like. You can even do it in two parts - the lists and then the visualization. (Why not drop me a message to tell me how it went?)

one
Write a list of five things you've been holding yourself back from doing because of your body hang-ups or because you haven't got your dream body yet.

Think about how your life would change if you could let go of this fantasy goal.

two
Next, write five things you would like to do more of if you could embrace the body you have right now. (Yeah baby, rolls and all.)

three
Now you've got your two lists - one list is what you're moving away from and one list is what you're moving toward. Time to let go of the fantasy body. I know, it's kinda painful, it may be emotional, but don't forget what we've learned so far. It doesn't mean giving up on being happy, fit and healthy. It's just about ridding yourself of a vision of yourself that's likely unrealistic and makes you feel bad.

four

Ok, so find somewhere quiet and close your eyes.
Think about the things that are holding you back and
then, in your mind, turn them black and white and make
them smaller and smaller. Think about the dream body
you've been measuring yourself up against and also begin
to make this version of yourself smaller and black and
white, until it's almost disappeared.

five

Now begin to think about all the things you want to do
more of. Make them brighter, more colourful and fill your
mind. Block out the black and white images with these
colourful ones. See yourself as you are now, but living
your best life doing all the things you want to do more of.

Bring the feeling of having found this new love of
yourself into your body as you sit there.

six

Say goodbye to the fantasy (blow her a kiss as you
make her disappear) because the joy you feel in yourself
in this technicolour reality is way, way better. Smile
(actually) because you've found ways to feel happy
and healthy that don't involve the guilt and shame
that the old fantasy body used to give you.

seven

When you're ready, come back into the space and write
a few notes about the feeling. Use this visualization
to motivate you further on this path.

tips

Whatever comes up, no judgement. It's all part of the healing.
Do everything with curiosity and compassion. Stop as much
as you need. And explore how it feels to show yourself
some kindness.

★ SUMMARY ★

+ BODY NEUTRALITY IS AN IMPORTANT STEP IN MAKING PEACE WITH YOUR BODY.

+ YOUR BODY HEARS EVERYTHING YOUR BRAIN TELLS IT.

+ BUT... YOU DON'T HAVE TO CARRY AROUND NEGATIVE THOUGHTS ABOUT YOURSELF.

+ YOU ARE AS MUCH YOUR THIGHS AS YOUR EYES.

+ YOU HAVE EVERYTHING INSIDE YOURSELF TO LEARN TO EAT INTUITIVELY.

+ EATING THIS WAY TAKES PATIENCE AND PRACTICE - STAY SUPER KIND TO YOURSELF.

+ YOU HAVE TO GIVE UP YOUR "FANTASY BODY", BUT WHEN YOU DO YOU'RE READY TO CREATE A NEW REALITY AND YOU'RE WELL ON THE PATH TO FREEDOM.

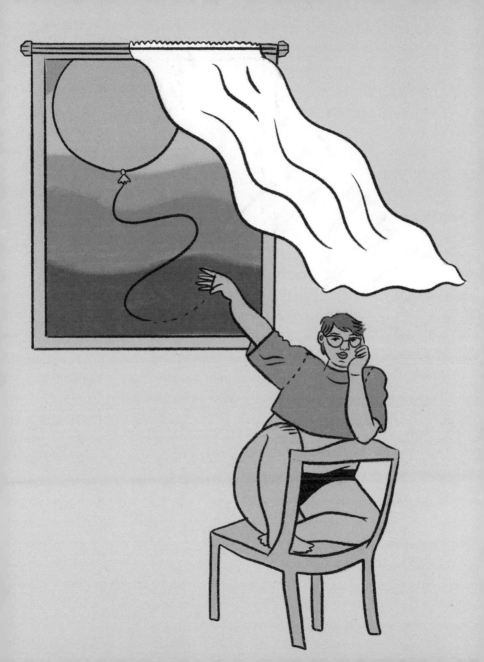

MYTHS, DEMONS & THE END OF THE YELLOW BRICK ROAD

As we wander further up our Yellow Brick Road, we're likely to come across some stumbling blocks (remember how Dorothy had to overcome those terrifying flying monkeys?).

I'm going to talk a lot about being kind to yourself in the face of these adversaries. So let's work on how this feels. (If being kind to yourself feels alien to you, the Cultivating Kindness activity on page 85 is especially important.)

If you're ever in doubt as to how to act in a situation, I want you to tap into the "What would my bestie do?" mindset (WWMBD?!). It's with this way of thinking that you'll be able to cultivate kindness to yourself. The more you do this, the easier it gets.

Next on our journey to peaceful body mojo – myth busting.

There's some right nonsense out there when it comes to body acceptance. So it's time to level up your knowledge and your skills so you can slay whatever potential challengers (or demons) come your way when you're out in the world.

LET'S GO.

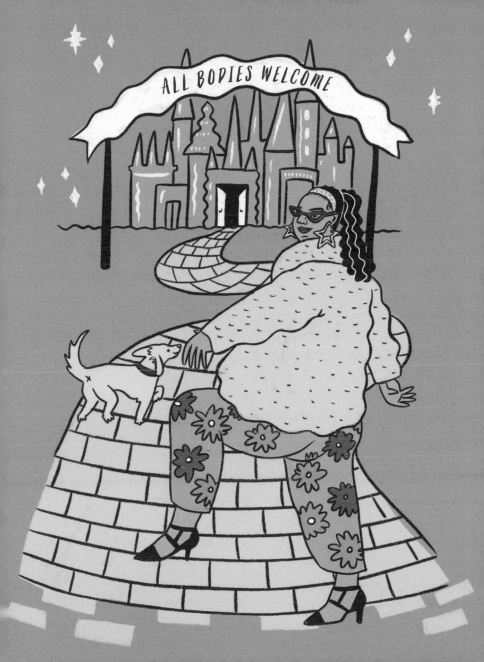

FAT IS NOT A FEELING (& WHY CURIOSITY IS SO ACE)

How many times have you exclaimed to yourself, be it out loud or just inside your mind, "I feel fat"? Hundreds of times? A thousand?

Well hunny, fat is not a feeling, it's a descriptor.

I have fat. Just like I have green eyes, fingernails and, in my case, bleached AF hair.

We all have fat. We would die without it. Yet those three words are some of the most loaded we have in our back pocket. I know just too well how the words "I feel fat" can turn a nice time into a weeping nightmare.

I remember how, as a teenager in particular but through my twenties too, the task of getting ready to go out could easily end in exasperated tears. I'd cover my room with item after item of dismissed clothing, a rising sense of despair and the sensation of "fatness" getting ever more intense.

And what about a good ol' fashioned changing room moment?

There's nothing like taking a huge armful of clothes to the changing room and not managing to get ANY of the five pairs of jeans that had looked nice on the rack up over your thighs*. Suddenly the lights are too bright, there's sweat on your brow and a sinking feeling in your heart. I. Feel. Your. Pain.

(*Or tops buttoned over your boobs. Or arm holes that are too tight. Or when you fear you might be stuck in the dress. Or when things are hanging off you in such a bizarre way that you think there must be something wrong with your body.)

But it's not your fault! We are conditioned to blame (and shame) our bodies instead of looking at the bigger picture and working out what's really going on.

> I WANT TO REITERATE THIS IMPORTANT POINT: FAT ISN'T A BAD WORD. WE USE IT AS THE WORST THING WE CAN SAY ABOUT OURSELVES, BUT THIS DOESN'T HAVE TO BE THE CASE.

I'd like to invite you to consider how it would feel to reclaim the word "fat" as a descriptor, and therefore take back its power. (I promise, it really doesn't need to have the devastating impact that we so often feel it does.) There are now heaps of women who have reclaimed the word "fat". They're loudly and proudly declaring themselves "fat babes" in an empowered, loving way, and it's awesome.

I'm not saying that you have to do the same. It is entirely up to each person how they want to engage with the word "fat". But I want you to know that it doesn't have to be the worst thing you (or someone else) can say about yourself.

Telling ourselves that we feel fat in such a negative way (not only is it inherently fat-phobic) but we're using it as emotional self-harm.

> WE'RE NOT ONLY TELLING OURSELVES THAT WE'RE NOT GOOD ENOUGH, BUT WE'RE OFTEN ALSO NEGLECTING TO FEEL OUR FEELINGS PROPERLY.

I guarantee that every time I've ever said it in my life, I could replace the word "fat" with something else much more real to the situation. How about the words "sad", "scared", "vulnerable", "angry", "insecure" or "unlovable"? Those would probably cover most of it.

VERY IMPORTANT SIDE NOTE[*]

I feel that it's fair to say that whatever word you're using negatively against your body can be covering up how you really feel. However, if examining your feelings is bringing up any sort of trauma or is too difficult to deal with on your own, please find local support (therapy is awesome and should be shouted about).

Ok, so now we've established that we're bypassing what's really going on and blaming our bodies. Here's a super useful tool for getting rid of this nasty judgement.

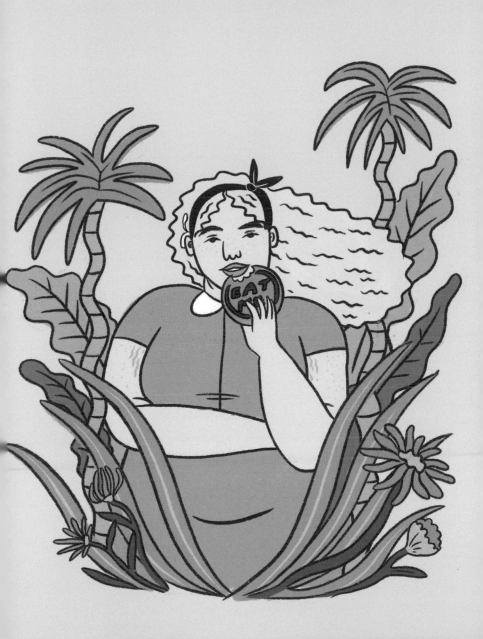

CURIOSITY

"Curiouser and curiouser", said Alice after she'd eaten the cake marked "Eat me" (like any food lover would). And while Alice started to grow into a GIANT, she managed not to blame herself (or freak out) but simply invoke the power of curiosity.

Curiosity is awesome. It's something that's inherent in all of us. We all know what it feels like to be inquisitive as children (many parents have been driven mad with "But whyyyyyy?").

This gets knocked out of us as adults, but it's going to become your new super power in the fight against negative thoughts and self-judgement. Why? (See, you're getting it already.) Because curiosity lets you become a detective* to learn about yourself. (*Detective hat not essential, but don't let me get in the way of a good accessory.)

> BY GETTING INTO THE HABIT OF TAKING SMALL MOMENTS TO REFLECT, IT CREATES SPACE BETWEEN YOU AND THE BEHAVIOUR OR THOUGHTS. THIS MEANS YOU CAN TAKE A STEP BACK AND BECOME AN OBSERVER TO THE SITUATION.

I believe any situation you'll come across in this journey of self-discovery and self-compassion can be used as an opportunity for discovery and growth.

Add to this new tool a dollop of kindness (like, a big one, like a child-let-loose-with-the-chocolate-sauce type deal), because we all need more kindness, always. Then we're in the mix for some magic... this is where we have to ask ourselves some questions to find out what's been happening.

Here are some examples of curiosity questions. Feel free to start with an inquisitive "Hhm... I wonder" while stroking your imaginary (or real) beard.

+ **WHY DID THAT HAPPEN?**

+ **WAS THERE A TRIGGER?**

+ **HOW WAS I FEELING BEFORE?**

+ **HOW DO I FEEL NOW?**

+ **WHAT DO I NEED RIGHT NOW?**

+ **HOW CAN I BE KINDER TO MYSELF IN THIS MOMENT?**

+ **AM I TRYING TO TELL MYSELF SOMETHING?**

When we're able to look at situations more fully (through developing curiosity) we get to see the emotions that are UNDER them and then we're able to treat the root cause of the issue instead of creating a feeling of failure or complete self-judgement.

Let's use an example. You've blindly eaten your way through an entire packet of chocolate cookies before the ad break is over. Doh! Before you fall into a spiral of self-hating thoughts about how you need a lock on the cupboard and should never be allowed to eat sugar again – Stop. Breathe. *Reflect*.

Ask yourself some curiosity questions... Why did that happen? Are you stressed? Are you trying to numb out? Are you tired? Do you feel unloved? Unseen? Unheard? Are you hanging on to some diet mentality that says you're not allowed to eat cookies? Do you need a conversation? A holiday? A hug? An early night? A night out? More support getting off diets?

> STOP DOING YOURSELF A MASSIVE DISSERVICE
> BY SUPPRESSING WHAT YOU ACTUALLY NEED.
> ASK YOURSELF, "HOW CAN I MAKE MYSELF
> FEEL BETTER?"

Sometimes, for me, "feeling fat" was actually my body craving movement and extra nourishment. I needed to make more loving choices toward myself – not punish myself with this bullying voice. We need to stop putting all our emotional happiness on our bodies.

Check out how by drilling down into your emotions. By being curious you can actually feel what you actually need! Our poor bodies, getting all the flack for all this other crap.

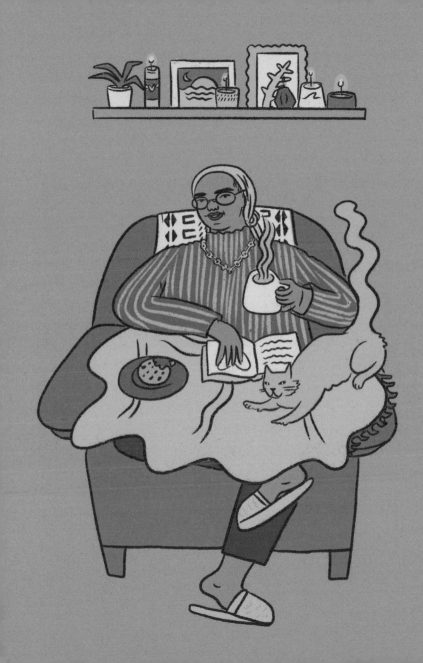

THIN-HEALTHY, FAT-UNHEALTHY

Next time you're hanging out on Instagram see if you spot any of these two types of photo.

Photo A is a thin, conventionally attractive woman eating a huge burger, the type you see in eating challenges (greasy, cheesy, meaty massiveness). She's taking a bite. Underneath, the comments probably go something like this, "Oh yeah! That looks so good", "That's so hot", "Mmm you go girl".

Photo B is a person exercising. They're sweating and smiling. But... their body is bigger. The comments (ugh, stay out of the comments) probably go something like this, "You shouldn't be seen in public like that", "Gross!", "Someone should tell her not to wear Lycra", "Stop eating!"

Now tell me, are people really concerned about someone's health when they're making those comments? I think not.

I would consider critically (and lovingly if they're your friend) the person banging the drum on health around other people's bodies. **Because, quite frankly, you cannot tell a person's health from looking at them.**

A person's weight doesn't tell you what they eat, how much they exercise, how strong they are. It doesn't tell you if they were once thinner or fatter. It doesn't tell you if they've battled an illness. In short, weight tells you f*** all about a person.

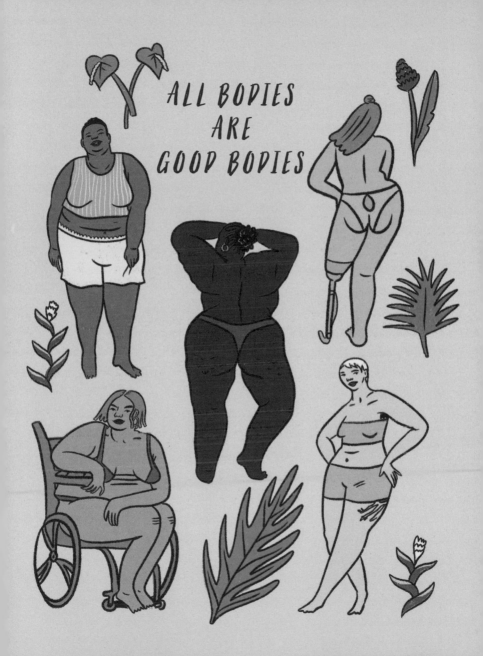

Here are six reasons why I call out "health" comments as "concern trolling".

one

Health is holistic and multifaceted. It's not simply about aesthetics, like a thin body. Health is about our habits and mentality (and is in no way a moral obligation, just fyi).

two

Health is greatly impacted by income and other socio-economic factors. What food we have access to and can afford is a f***ing big deal, which often gets overlooked.

three

Physical health is impacted by our mental health, which is often neglected, and health is judged on how we look physically. Self-esteem is a big player in our health. (*Shock news* telling someone that they're unhealthy isn't great for their self-esteem.)

four

Health is affected by the care we have access to (and the care we receive - see Fatphobia on pages 88-89).

five

Health is impacted by our genetics - something we have no control over.

six

Health exists in the complexity of our lives and identities. Put simply, health is not about weight. There are many papers that show that "health-promoting behaviours" (things like giving up smoking, eating enough fibre and moving more) are better determiners of health than weight.

For some bizarre reason, being "in good health" is held up as the pinnacle of existence. I'm calling that out as complete BS.

Hear me when I say: regardless of your size, how well your body functions or how "healthy" you are – you are allowed to love yourself. **You are worthy of love and respect simply for existing as a magical human being.** Your body deserves love and respect at any size and at any level of health. Forget societal health expectations, ableism, privilege and stereotypes, and forget anyone who tells you otherwise.

The debate on obesity is rife with conflicting research. I would urge you to always be aware of who is funding the research.

> THE MAIN TAKE AWAY I'D LIKE YOU, DEAR READER, TO GET FROM THIS IS AN UNDERSTANDING THAT IT IS POSSIBLE TO BE FAT AND HAPPY AND HEALTHY. JUST AS IT'S POSSIBLE TO BE THIN AND UNHEALTHY.

Just dip into Instagram and see the number of beautiful bigger bodies being bendy yogis, vegans, runners and all manner of "wellness trait" persons, whose bodies remain where they are.

Judging someone by the size of their body is strictly visual, and it flattens that person into a meaningless number.

Cultivating kindness

Think about a time your best friend was there for you.
Maybe you were upset about a mean comment, a break-
up or a test you flunked. Maybe it was an event where
you felt silly, embarrassed or where you felt you let
someone down. It doesn't matter what the situation was.

one
Take a moment to remember the moment
(yuck, it's slimy again, I feel you).

two
Think about the words your friend said or might have said
to soothe you. These might be things like "I'm sorry that
happened to you", "It wasn't your fault", "You're not a bad
person", "You're only human", "You're lovely just the way
you are" or "F*** what others think".

three
Write them down. Look at the list and think about how
they make you feel. If you can, read them out loud and
try to really hear them. These words are for you. How
does that make you feel?

four
See if you can let them soften you, soothe you and
take a moment to feel their kindness toward you.
The more we do this, the easier it becomes to use
the same voice for ourselves.

HEALTH AT EVERY SIZE

This is where I'm so grateful that Health At Every Size®
(HAES) exists. It's a movement created by Linda Bacon that
"supports people of all sizes in finding compassionate ways
of taking care of themselves". HAES removes weight from the
health equation and looks at other markers for health. And
it's these healthy habits that are the most important factors
when looking at health, and they're what we should all be
focusing on and encouraging (not the pursuit of weight loss).

HAES has three pillars, which much of my teaching is based on:

+ **BODY RESPECT AND CELEBRATING BODY DIVERSITY**
  (ALL bodies are good bodies!).

+ **CRITICAL THINKING ABOUT SCIENTIFIC AND CULTURAL
  ASSUMPTIONS**
  (bias and opinions need outing when looking at science).

+ **COMPASSIONATE SELF-CARE**
  (this includes moving in a way that feels good, and eating in
  an intuitive way).

Go and buy the book (see Further Reading on page 111)
because it will blow your mind on this subject and really help
you on your next stage of your journey.

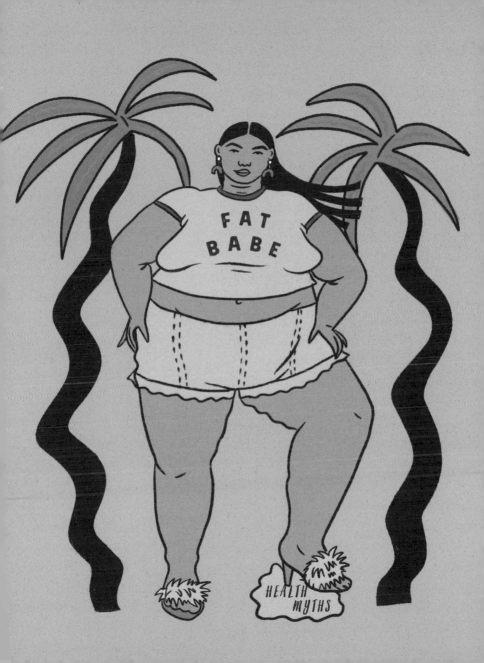

FATPHOBIA

The fear of fatness and the way that people in bigger bodies are negatively treated and labelled is called fatphobia.

As a result of this normalized culture of stigma and shame, people in bigger bodies continuously have to think about how to protect themselves. They must negotiate, or avoid completely, situations that other people take for granted.

Things like: avoiding gyms and other places of exercise, going home late at night on public transport on their own, worrying about getting on planes and eating in public. Not only that, but there is a serious weight bias in the healthcare industry that leads to people being discriminated against, misdiagnosed or not given the treatment they need. Consequently, many fat people avoid going to the doctor altogether because of the fear of being shamed.

I really hate to go back to the woes of society (we left that dark place earlier in the book), but knowing that this is the reality for some people (or perhaps yourself) is important in understanding your relationship with your body.

If you're living in a thin body, please take a moment to appreciate the privileges that come with it because many people are facing daily battles just existing in the world. See Further Reading on pages 110–111 for some books written by incredible babes giving two fingers to fatphobic discrimination.

In diet culture, the fear of "being fat and unhealthy" is meant to motivate us to stay continuously working toward the golden ticket of living *ding ding* thin and healthy.

BUT IS IT ACTUALLY WORKING?

Hell no, it isn't. Diets and discrimination aren't making us thinner and they sure aren't making us happier. It's really hard to accept (and definitely love) your body when we live in a society that so openly hates fatness. Don't let this depress you, loves. Remember those rebel attitudes? We need them now because, for all the reasons listed above, this is not ok!

SELF-CARE CHECK-IN...

How are you feeling after learning about fatphobia? Check in and see what you're feeling right now.

If it's triggered some painful memories about discrimination you've experienced, feel free to stop reading now and do something that will make you feel better. If it's all new to you, does it make you think a bit differently about your own experience? This is a pit stop to say that you have permission to feel how you feel. Journal, call a friend, take your dog for a walk, take five, write an angry letter (but don't post it yet), watch an old episode of something funny, hug your knees, breathe. **Do what you need to do.**

YOU'LL NEVER HAVE A BAD DAY AGAIN

Oh how I wish this were true! Even as far along as I am in my journey, there are still days when I'm not my own best friend. There are still times I catch myself wishing away things like cellulite (even though it's entirely NORMAL, damn you diet culture) and imagining what it must be like to look different.

Diet culture is everywhere. You're allowed to think it's too hard some days, because it is super hard! We live in a society that is designed to make us feel bad about ourselves.

The difference for me from then to now, though, is that I DON'T allow those thoughts to rule my life any more. If I'm "feeling fat", I use curiosity questions to assess what I need. I call out diet culture and I edit my social media feeds so that they're places I want to hang out. (Do this. It's so powerful.)

My mental recovery from woe to "wow (you look good!)" is much shorter and my emotional resilience is way stronger. I promise, the more you practise, the easier you'll find it too.

VERY IMPORTANT SIDE NOTE

Please throw away your scales. Scales are a poor determiner of weight. They only tell you the gravitational pull you're having to the planet. They don't consider water weight or if you're carrying a food baby (or a big poo, sorrynotsorry!). They are GUARANTEED to make you feel 10 x worse on a bad day. I suggest posting a photo of smashed-up scales (#riotsnotdiets) and recycling that piece of junk.

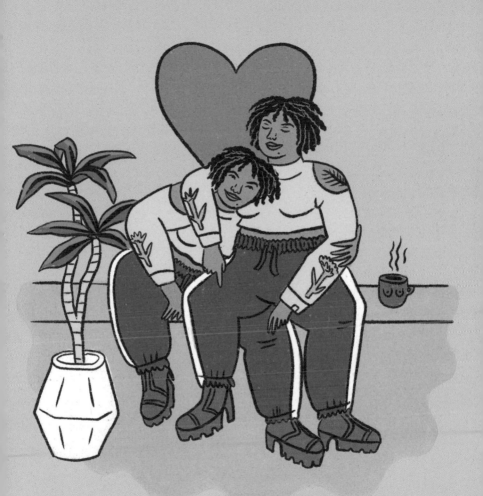

YOU CAN BE YOUR
OWN BEST FRIEND

YOU'LL SIT ON THE SOFA ALL DAY

Do you know what's really cool about getting rid of diet mentality and gaining body acceptance? You start wanting to do more nice things that make you feel good – and this quite possibly involves healing your relationship with exercise. (Don't close the pages! I promise I'm not about to sneak a personal training plan on you.)

Stop thinking of exercise as a way to lose weight and start thinking of it solely as a way to feel good.

+ No more pressure to keep up habits you hate.

+ No more doing it "because it's good for you".

+ No more feeling like a failure.

How awesome does that sound?

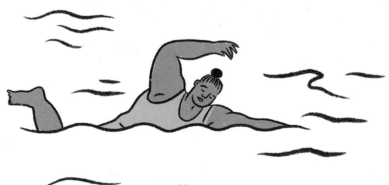

Movement as medicine

one

Taking away a goal weight or target, think about how you
would like to **feel** in your body in the next three months. What
words would you use to describe this new sensation? Maybe
more alive, lighter, more energetic, less tired, less achy, freer,
more subtle, less tight, refreshed, zingy, relaxed, stronger,
happier, less out of breath, more alert?

Go ahead, take five minutes and write down some words.

two

Ok, now how would you like your body
to feel next month?

three

And finally, how would you like your body
to feel next week?

four

What type of movement (remember, these only have
to be baby steps) could you try out next week, next month
and in the next three months to incorporate these feelings
into your life?

five

Make a promise to yourself to try it and vow
to keep that promise as if you were making it
to your dearest loved one.

EXERCISE DOES NOT NEED TO BE PUNISHMENT

Exercise is simply movement. Moving your body is good for you. Duh! I'm not about to tell you the benefits of exercise (although there are tons, from happier hearts to more sound sleeps). How you choose to move your body is up to you.

But the fact of the matter is, we're not doing enough of it. And in my experience, it's because we think that in order to "exercise properly", we must be doing it in some formalized manner, like going to the gym (with goals and PBs) or taking a spin class or hitting the yoga mat at 6am, preferably wearing some fancy matching Lycra. This is the "wellness" curse!

MOVEMENT CAN BE WHATEVER YOU WANT IT TO BE - IT DOES NOT MATTER IF IT'S GENTLE WALKING, FOOTBALL, ULTIMATE FRISBEE, CAN-CAN DANCING, MOSHING IN YOUR KITCHEN OR HOPSCOTCH WITH YOUR KIDS (OR YOUR FRIENDS FOR THAT MATTER). PLAY AS MUCH AS YOU CAN.

It can be at home in your sports bra and knickers or out in the wilds. It can be on your own, in a team, with your pet, with your partner or with complete strangers. There is no need to publicly exercise if you do not want to.

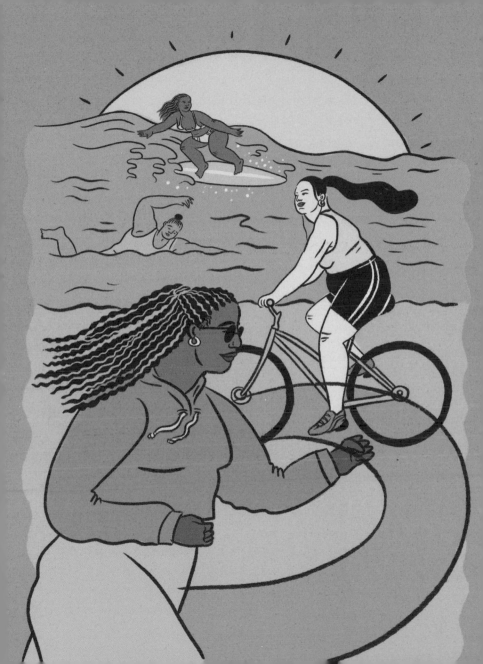

**Exercise should nourish you and make your body sing.
It doesn't need to destroy you.**

When you take away the imagined goal and focus on the
FEELING – you get to move in a way that simply makes you
feel that way. So, if you're stressed AF at work – you might
want to try yoga to relax you. Or if you're feeling sluggish,
then why not get outdoors and blow those cobwebs away.

I promise, the more you explore and move from a place
of curiosity and kindness (sorrynotsorry to keep going on
about this dynamo duo), then you'll really not want to sit on
the sofa all day, because you'll be free of expectations and
feelings of failure and high on how movement makes you feel.

Ok, so can you commit to the following promise for me?

MOVEMENT PROMISE

"I, [your name], promise to explore movement from a place
of how it makes me feel. I promise to remove judgement of
how good I am at it. I promise to do it with an open mind.
I promise not to think about any other goal apart from
to check in with my feelings afterward. And I promise, if
this movement isn't "doing it" for me I'll try another one –
because there are infinite ways I can move my body."

NOTHING TASTES AS GOOD AS SKINNY FEELS – OH WAIT, ACTUALLY TONS DOES!

You've probably heard the famous Kate Moss quote "nothing tastes as good as skinny feels". It is said in a way that keeps us in check every time we want to eat a mouthful of cake. Like "fridge pickers wear big knickers" and "a moment on the lips, a lifetime on the hips" (two more expressions that send me into a quiet rage when I hear people use them).

I'd like to shine a light on this particular toxic piece of advice because, quite frankly, I've had enough of it.

BODY ACCEPTANCE FEELS AND TASTES BETTER THAN SKINNY FEELS.

Remember when I told you that acceptance is NOT GIVING UP. This is because there's so much freedom in learning to love your body. Let's explore this further.

There's the **physical** freedom as you can live your life free from insecurities. And there's also the **mental** freedom as you have so much more brain space for other things.

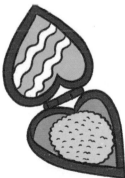

Here are seven things I think taste better than skinny feels:

one

MORE ADVENTURE. Making peace with your body so you no longer feel like you're waiting for your life to start in a mythical place in the future "when...I've lost 10lbs". More fun times NOW.

two

MORE SUNSHINE ON SKIN. Wearing whatever you want regardless of what magazines say and choosing clothes that make you happy not because you think they flatter you.

three

MORE STRUTS. Instead of a towel shuffle, you're free to shimmy down the beach with your head held high. Or strut down the street giving yourself a wink in the shop window (hi gorgeous one!). I give you permission to think that you're cute AF.

four

MORE TIME FOR LIVING. Imagine the joy of saying "why not?"
when people ask you to try new things (like pottery class, learning
Korean or mastering the perfect loaf) because you've got rid of
all the obsessive thoughts about food and your body that used
to take up so much brain space.

five

MORE LIVING BY YOUR OWN RULES. Saying a mental goodbye
to diet culture and anyone who says you have to change your
body to be happy.

six

MORE LOVE (AND KEEPING THE LIGHT ON). Insecurities stop us from feeling
attractive to others. I want you to know that you're super sexy to
someone! And you deserve to have as much love (and sexy times!)
as anyone else.

seven

MORE GRATITUDE. Your body is amazing. Appreciate every
hug, smile, kiss and breath.

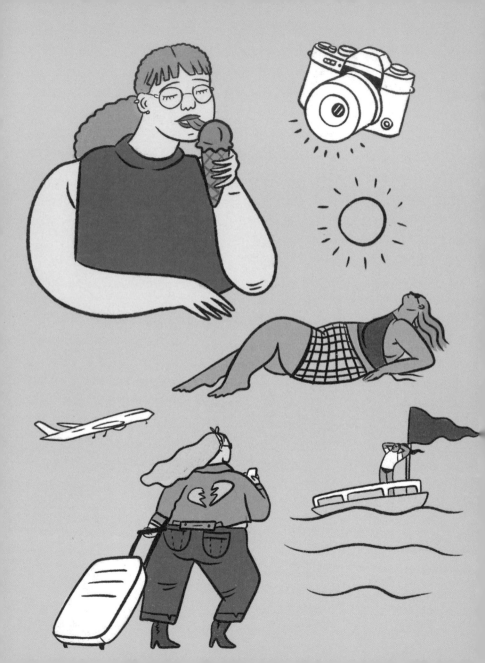

Write twenty things you think will taste better than
skinny feels:

*
*
*
*
*
*
*
*
*
*
*
*
*
*
*
*
*
*
*
*

★ SUMMARY ★

+ THERE WILL BE BUMPS ON THE ROAD, BUT ARMED
  WITH ENOUGH KNOWLEDGE, YOU'LL BE ABLE TO FACE
  DOWN THE DEMONS AND THE HATERS.

+ FAT IS NOT A FEELING - USE CURIOSITY QUESTIONS
  TO FIND OUT WHAT YOUR BODY REALLY NEEDS.

+ FAT DOESN'T AUTOMATICALLY MEAN UNHEALTHY. WE
  HAVE TO CHECK OUR ASSUMPTIONS AROUND WHAT
  PEOPLE LOOK LIKE AND THEIR HEALTH.

+ LEARNING TO ACCEPT YOUR BODY IS HARD - THERE'LL
  STILL BE BAD DAYS, BUT YOU'LL DEVELOP MORE
  RESILIENCE ON YOUR PATH.

+ BODY ACCEPTANCE GIVES YOU THE MENTAL AND
  PHYSICAL FREEDOM TO EXPERIENCE ALL OF THE GREAT
  BOUNTIES THAT LIFE HAS TO OFFER.

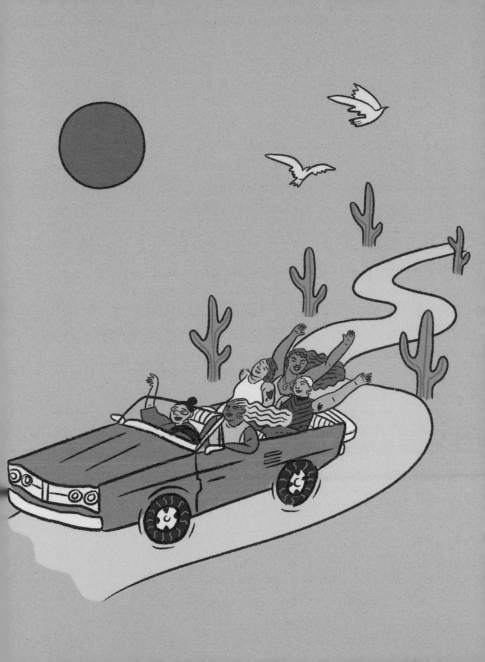

THERE'S NO PLACE LIKE HOME (FINDING YOUR RUBY SLIPPERS)

We've taken a whistle-stop tour of the world of diet culture, how we eat, health and body acceptance myths – what a roller coaster. By now I hope you're starting to feel that treating yourself like your best friend is possible, or at least coming round to a gentler way of thinking. My biggest hope is that you see how getting off diets can lead to a happier mental place.

The more you can understand the world we live in and how the messages we're fed daily destroy our self-esteem, the more you can cultivate kindness (get rid of your inner bitch) and discover what your body really wants. And the more you'll heal your relationship with your body.

Healing your relationship with your body (and with food) is not linear. It is, in fact, very bumpy. But I hope you'll start to see that it's worth it. That you're worth it.

Now is a good time to look back at the answers you gave to the questions on page 13. Can you push any of your ratings further up the scale toward 10 (meaning "all the yes")? Even if you only move each up by 1, that's improvement baby!

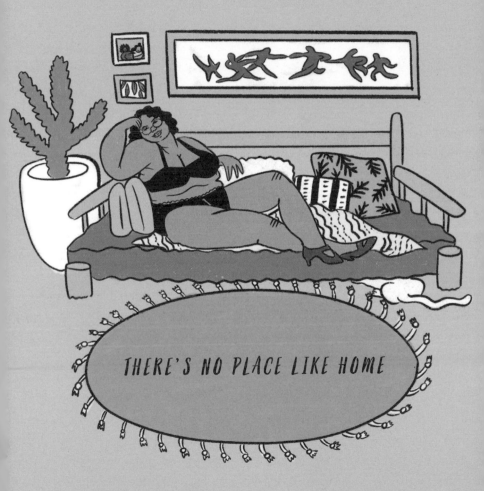
THERE'S NO PLACE LIKE HOME

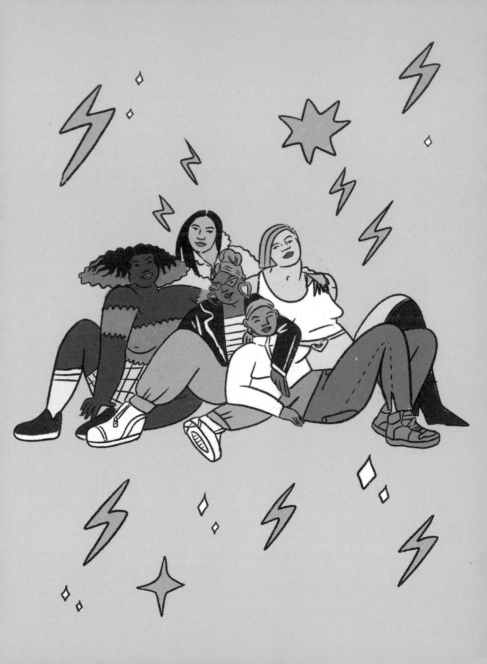

ANY STEP TOWARD LOVING YOURSELF SHOULD
BE CELEBRATED.

In my coaching practice, *it's all about celebrating the small wins.* Treat yourself to something you wouldn't normally... it doesn't have to be buying something (although it does feel nice sometimes). It could be taking yourself to your favourite place. Having a pamper evening at home. Or cooking yourself something you really, really fancy now you're starting to listen more to what your body needs (woop!).

SO WHAT NEXT?

Dr Kristin Neff is the queen of self-compassion. She says something that I feel is incredibly important.

She says: "Instead of mercilessly judging and criticizing yourself for various inadequacies or shortcomings, self-compassion means you are kind and understanding when confronted with personal failings – after all, whoever said you were supposed to be perfect? You may try to change in ways that allow you to be more healthy and happy, but this is done because you care about yourself, not because you are worthless or unacceptable as you are."

This to me is body-loving nirvana – and this is what I want for you.

There is no such thing as a perfect body. There really are no such things as "flaws" either. There is no such thing as the perfect diet. Or perfect eating. You don't need shrinking, fixing or changing. These are further myths we're sold.

What is real is that you are unique. You are a living, breathing, bundle of scientific magic. It's so cliched to say "there's only one of you" but that's the truth!

You are you. And truly, that's enough.

IN A WORLD THAT'S HARD, SIMPLY BEING KIND TO YOURSELF IS A REBELLIOUS ACT.

Your body shape has never had, or ever will have, anything to do with how much happiness, or how much love, you can have in the world. And the more you can become your greatest ally, the easier it is to finally embrace the skin you're in (you'll finally get your very own pair of ruby red slippers).

Life is yours for the taking – give everything that tells you otherwise the middle finger and go out and take it. You can be your own crush.

I BELIEVE IN YOU.

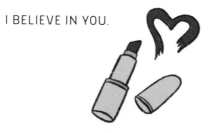

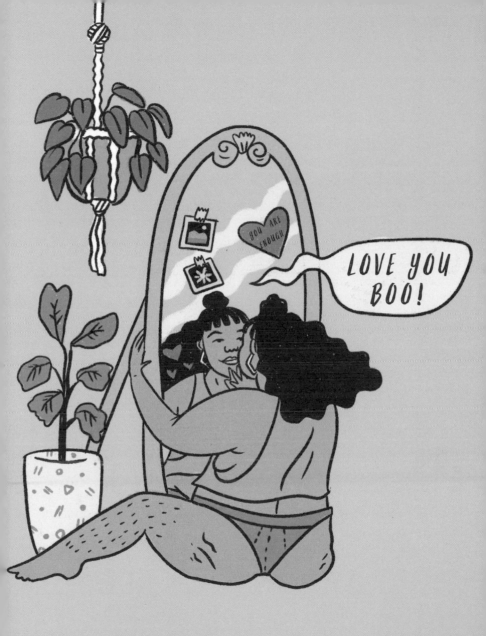

★ FURTHER READING ★

This is a list of books I think will help you build knowledge of the subjects we've covered within these pages, plus some personal stories I think you'll enjoy.

Ann Saffi Biasetti, *Befriending Your Body: A Self-Compassionate Approach to Freeing Yourself from Disordered Eating* (Shambhala Publications Inc, 2018)

Brené Brown, *Daring Greatly* (Penguin Life, 2015)

Ellyn Satter, *Ellyn Satter's Secrets of Feeding a Healthy Family: How to Eat, How to Raise Good Eaters, How to Cook* (Kelcy Press, 2008)

Evelyn Tribole, M.S., R.D. and Elyse Resch, M.S., R.D., F.A.D.A., *Intuitive Eating: A Revolutionary Program That Works,* revised edition (St. Martin's Griffin, 2012)

Geneen Roth, *Breaking Free from Emotional Eating* (Plume, 2004)

Harriet Brown, *Body of Truth: How Science, History, and Culture Drive Our Obsession with Weight – and What We Can Do about It* (Da Capo Press, 2015)

Jes Baker, *Things No One Will Tell Fat Girls: A Handbook for Unapologetic Living* (Seal Press, 2015)

Laura Fraser, *Losing it: America's Obsession with Weight and the Industry That Feeds on it* (Dutton, 1997)

Laura Thomas PhD, *Just Eat It* (Bluebird, 2019)

Linda Bacon and Lucy Aphramor, *Body Respect: What Conventional Health Books Get Wrong, Leave Out, and Just Plain Fail to Understand about Weight* (BenBella, 2014)

Linda Bacon, *Health At Every Size: The Surprising Truth About Your Weight* (BenBella, 2010)

Megan Crabbe, *Body Positive Power: How to stop dieting, make peace with your body and live* (Vermilion, 2017)

Michelle Elman, *Am I Ugly?* (Anima, 2018)

Naomi Wolf, *The Beauty Myth: How Images of Beauty are Used Against Women* (Vintage Classics, 2015)

Ruby Tandoh, *Eat Up* (Serpent's Tail, 2018)

Sarai Walker, *Dietland: a wickedly funny, feminist revenge fantasy novel of one fat woman's fight against sexism and the beauty industry* (Atlantic Books, 2016)

★ RESOURCES ★

BEAT: The UK's Eating Disorder Charity 0808 801 0677
National Eating Disorders Association Helpline (US) 1-800-931-2237
Mind (UK mental health charity) 0300 123 3393
Mental Health America 1-800-273-TALK (8255)

Health at Every Size https://haescommunity.com
Ellyn Satter Institute www.EllynSatterInstitute.org

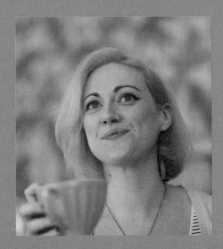

HARRI ROSE IS A QUALIFIED HEALTH COACH AND MINDFULNESS TEACHER. SHE TEACHES BODY ACCEPTANCE, SELF-COMPASSION AND CREATIVE LIVING. HARRI BELIEVES THAT FOR TOO LONG WE HAVE BEEN APOLOGIZING FOR OUR BODIES - AND THAT DIET CULTURE AND BEAUTY STANDARDS ARE HOLDING US BACK. THROUGH HER WRITING, WORKSHOPS AND 1:1 CLIENTS, HARRI HELPS PEOPLE TO LIVE THEIR LIVES WITHOUT RULES AND RESTRICTION AND EMBRACE HOW AMAZING THEY REALLY ARE.

FIND HER ON INSTAGRAM @HARRI_ROSE_ OR AT HER WEBSITE HARRIROSE.COM